Leather And Latex Care

Leather And Latex Care

How To Keep Your Leather And Latex Looking Great

Kelly J. Thibault

Daedalus Publishing
2140 Hyperion Avenue
Los Angeles, CA 90027

This trade paperback is published by

Daedalus Publishing
2140 Hyperion Avenue,
Los Angeles, CA 90027
www.daedaluspublishing.com

Library of Congress Catalog Card Number: 95-80430

ISBN: 1-881943-00-3

Manufactured in the United States of America

Dedication

This book is dedicated to Mom, Dad, Cathy, Jeff, Persephone, and Backdraft to help honor their unconditional love.

Table of Contents

Introduction 9

The History Of Leather 11

The Tanning Process 15

Basic Care For Leather 23

Helpful Leather Care Hints 31

A Short History Of Rubber 43

The Processing Of Raw Latex Rubber 49

The Care Of Latex Garments 53

Conclusion 61

About The Author 63

INTRODUCTION

As a member of the Leather community, I am constantly amazed at the number of people who really don't know how to care properly for the object of their affection, their leathers, and in some cases their latex. Whether you are a seasoned warrior or a novice to the leather lifestyle, this book is intended to help you give your leather possessions the care they need to ensure a long life and a beautiful appearance. Some may fear that this is a complicated task, but it need not be. On the contrary, anyone familiar with the household-tips column *Hints From Heloise* will be right at home. Most of what you will read about leather is knowledge I gained from my father, a former cowboy cobbler, and my uncle, a saddle maker. Both have extensive experience working with leather in their respective shops in Montana. Some of the procedures I have discovered myself through trial and error, including most of what is known about latex. I would like to emphasize that this care guide is just that—a guide. It is not the definitive word on leather and latex care, but is a general manual meant to be easy to use. As with most tasks, there is always more than one acceptable way to reach the goal. With this in mind, I hope you find the book informative and as much fun to read as it was to write.

DISCLAIMER

I must also include, for the protection of myself and anyone associated with this book, the following disclaimer. This book contains some information that may unsettle some members of the general public. The information contained about contamination of leather or latex by body fluids is intended to help ward off unwanted disease transmission. While all information is aimed at keeping leather, latex, and our bodies in tip-top condition, everyone must take responsibility for his or her own actions. Therefore, the information contained in this book in not warrantied. Responsibility for the use of this information and its results rest solely with the reader.

THE HISTORY OF LEATHER

For primitive societies, learning to make leather was a key step in basic survival. Groups with such diverse anthropological backgrounds as the Eskimos, Native Americans and Africans used animal hide as raw material in the production of clothing, shelter, transportation and self-defense.

Early man found that hides could be made more durable by curing them. This process involved treating the skin by rubbing it with fat and then smoking it over a wood fire. Later, tannic acid found in various plant materials was used to preserve the hides.

Preserved decorative leather goods have been discovered in Egyptian tombs dating back to 1300 B.C. The Egyptian use of leather is not surprising, considering that the methodology for mummification and leather tanning are similar. However, the Chinese are thought to have used animal skins even earlier, curing their leather with a mixture of salts (alum) and mud. The Chinese are also thought to have been the first to use leather for decorative purposes, as evidenced by screens, boxes and other ornately decorated pieces.

The Greeks and Romans also developed leather as a craft. Principal to their credit is the art of book making. However, it was the Hebrews who discovered the precursor of modern oak bark tanning. They soaked animal skins in fermented oak bark, naturally high in tannic acid (or tannins). This process not only prevented the decomposition of the skin, but also made the resulting leather stronger and more pliable. It should be noted that leather cured by this process is the only type that works well for tooling or carving.

Morocco became a capital of leathercraft, handing secrets for working with leather down generation to generation. With Moroccan influence, the Spaniards used leather in a more decorative sense. They subjected leather to many decorative processes such as: applique, inlaying, stamping, and carving. We have all heard of Cordovan leather named after Cordova, Spain, the Spanish leather center. This type of leather is produced from horsehide. In the rest of Europe during the Middle Ages, craft guilds, including those for leather, were responsible for ensuring quality workmanship. In 1397, the Fraternity of Leatherworkers was organized.

While the Europeans were using leather for decorative purposes, Native Americans used leather for more practical purposes. Using buffalo hide, they fashioned moccasins, tents, leather laces and tomahawks. They also developed their own tanning process to make buckskin, a soft, flexible, water-resistant leather. The process involved removing hair and excess meat by soaking in a lye solution (made from ashes), scraping the skin, and drying them over slow-burning fires.

Early colonists learned the utility of leather from the Native Americans. With this new knowledge, they used it to fashion such useful items as: clothing, buckets, door coverings and hinges. Saddles were then produced from this material as these people moved west. In the beginning of the 19th Century, Sir Humphrey Davy experimented with the tanning process and discovered that tanning agents were found in a variety of trees besides oak. His experimentation lead to the discovery of modern chrome tanning by Augustus Schultz, an American chemist.

Today, leather has as many uses as you can possibly imagine. We all know where that can lead us.

THE TANNING PROCESS

The skin from a dead animal that is to be processed into leather is referred to as a pelt or hide. Once the animal dies, rapid decomposition begins, due in part to bacterial growth, unless stopped by the tanning process. There are several steps to this process, outlined below.

The first step in the production of leather is *curing*. This slows decomposition until the hide can undergo further processing. The most common form of curing is the treatment of the hide with salt (sodium chloride). This is accomplished in two ways; by spreading salt crystals on the hide (wet salting) or by soaking the pelt in a brine solution. The latter is a faster method and is used more in commercial leather production. Most bacteria responsible for decomposition are unable to live in this environment so the hide does not begin to rot.

When the pelt arrives at a tannery it is trimmed and sorted to fit into the tanning machinery. The pelts are then soaked in water containing chemical wetting agents. This restores some of the moisture lost from the pelt during the curing process. It also helps to further wash the hide.

After the moisture has been restored, special machinery with rollers and blades is used to remove excess fat, muscle, and flesh from the inside of the pelt. This is referred to as *fleshing*. On the opposite side of the pelt, the hair is still attached and usually is removed before further processing. (Fur production from small animals is an exception and a different process.) Removal of this hair is accomplished by a combination of chemical and mechanical processes. First, the pelts are soaked in a lime solution. The alkaline environment destroys the hair and attacks the roots so the hair will come free from the pelt. This also helps to loosen the epidermis (the outer layer of tough skin which hides the grain) and removes other soluble skin proteins. Finally, a machine is used to mechanically scrape the loosened hair from the hide. American Indians used animal bones as tools for performing these last two chores.

After the hair is removed, the residual chemical

depilatory agent must be removed. This occurs in three stages. First, the hides are washed in water, the pH (a measure of the amount of acid or base present) is adjusted to neutral, and they are treated with ammonium chloride or ammonium sulphate to convert the residual lime to a soluble compound that can be washed out. *Bating*, treatment with digestive enzymes, then occurs. The hides are then washed thoroughly.

Next, the hides are transferred to an acidic solution. This lowers the pH of the hide so the tanning process can occur. Tanning can't take place at high (alkaline) pH. The most common chemicals used for this process are salt and sulfuric acid. The process is called *pickling*.

Once the hide has reached an acidic pH, it is now ready for the actual tanning process. There are three methods of tanning commonly used: *chrome tanning*, *vegetable tanning*, and *oil tanning*. I will briefly describe each of these methods.

Chrome tanning is the most commonly used method in modern commercial tanning, primarily because of the speed with which a hide can be tanned. The hide is soaked in a revolving drum in a solution of chromium salts. The most often used salt is chromium sulfate. Leather which has been tanned by this method is nearly water-proof and is also stretchable.

Vegetable tanning, also known as bark tanning, most closely matches the procedures followed by the

Hebrews. Plant material, primarily the woods oak, chestnut, and quebracho (from Argentina), is chopped up and boiled to produce a solution rich in tannic acid. The hides are then soaked for a period of time. This method, although time consuming, is still in popular use today, because it produces a moldable leather capable of undergoing other tooling processes. Leather, when produced by this method, will not stretch when dry, but can be molded when wet.

Oil tanning uses fish and animal oils to preserve the hide. Leather produced by this method is very soft and flexible. Oil tanned leather can also withstand repeated wetting. Chamois is the best example of leather tanned by this method.

After the tanning process is complete, several additional steps may be used to develop the finished leather product. Wringing (remember old-fashioned washing machines?) removes excess moisture left from the tanning process, preparing the leather for further treatment.

To give the leather a uniform thickness, it is split and shaved by machines equipped with huge blades arranged horizontally. The top layer yields leather that is termed "top grain." The lower layers, which have no grain, are called "splits." It is these layers which are used to produce suede.

At the option of the tanner, re-tanning by another method may occur to combine qualities imparted to the leather by the various tanning methods. For example, a tanner may wish to combine the flexibility produced with oil tanning with the water-proofing of chrome tanning. This process is much quicker than the primary tan, taking about two hours. After this is complete, the leather may be colored. Coloring used to be performed exclusively with aniline-type dye, derived from coal, in a rotating drum. The rotation is important in this process to ensure an even and deep penetration of the dye. It also helps to avoid streaking. Today, many different types of dyes exist with different characteristics. Acid dyes penetrate leather easily and are used to produce bright shades. Metallized dyes are used to produce leather with subdued or pastel shading. Direct dyes are used for surface dyeing only and produce deep shades. Basic dyes are also used for surface dyeing, but result in brilliant shades.

Fat-liquoring is the final wet chemical operation in the tanning process. Utilizing oils and other fatty substances from animals, along with vegetable products and minerals, it lubricates the leather fibers so that the leather will still be flexible after drying. In addition to ensuring the pliability of the leather, fat-liquoring also helps add to the tensile strength of the leather.

After the fat-liquoring process, the leather is considered completely tanned. That is to say, it will not undergo decomposition normally by bacteria. Although the hide is now considered leather, there are several dry operations which complete the final product. These processes may also develop special qualities in the leather.

The first step of the dry operations is *setting out.* A machine smooths the grain and stretches the leather, while compressing it to remove excess water. Even after this process, the leather will be about sixty percent water. The next step is to remove even more moisture by *drying.*

Once dried, the leather will contain about 10 percent water. This is an equilibrium for the leather. That is to say, the leather will lose water about as rapidly as it will absorb it, keeping the moisture content at about ten percent. Drying can be accomplished in one of three ways. In the first method, the leather is draped over a horizontal bar and allowed to dry, much like clothes on a clothesline. The leather may also be stretched over a frame and held in place, then dried slowly in a drying oven. The third process is called *pasting.* The leather is literally pasted on a stainless steel surface with starch paste and then dried in a drying oven.

At this point, leather is too hard and stiff to work with easily, so it must be conditioned. A fine mist of water is sprayed on the leather, which then sits overnight. This mist raises the moisture content of the leather to about 25 percent.

Now that the leather contains the correct moisture, it undergoes *staking.* In this process, machines pull and roll the leather, rendering it more pliable and workable. This step, in conjunction with fat-liquoring, determines the final firmness or softness of the leather.

The next step is purely cosmetic. In *buffing*, the grain side of the leather is mechanically sanded. This reduces the appearance of visual blemishes on the leather. These blemishes may be due to barbed wire scars, animal fights, etc. If the leather contains no blemishes, it is not buffed, and is termed "full grain leather."

BASIC CARE FOR LEATHER

Leather, like your skin, has pores that can trap dirt and grime. In order to keep it looking new, follow this simple but vital routine.

First, after you wear your leather gear, be sure and at least run a cloth over it before sticking it back in the closet. This helps keep dust and dirt off the hide. If not done, the dust and dirt accumulate in the pores and creases of leather. Over a long period, these small particles can rub much like fine-grit sandpaper, and cause your leather to lose its natural luster. Eventually, the finish will wear off and the dirt will get into the fibers of the leather, possibly causing it to split and crack. It will also make it increasingly more difficult to obtain a good shine.

Because I live in Southern California, I rarely have to worry about mud collecting on my boots or other leather items. Unfortunately, this is not the case in other parts of the world. Mud, unlike simple dust and dirt, does two obvious things to your leather—makes it dirty and makes it wet. When leather gets muddy, it must be cleaned as quickly as possible. However, don't be too hasty. That is to say, do not put the article in question anywhere too hot—a clothes dryer or the sun, for example, if used to dry leather, will almost invariably shrink and possibly split the leather. The amount of shrinkage depends on the type of leather, and the tanning process used. For example, glove leather will shrink more than latigo. Leather that is tanned with acid will shrink more than that tanned with oil. Shrinkage can then cause the leather fibers to split.

To clean a muddy item, first use a soft broom or a cloth to remove most of the muck. Store the item in an out-of-the-way place while it dries slowly. Once the residual mud has dried, use a stiff brush to remove it from the leather. Any stiff brush, except of course one made of wire, will work for this task. I typically use a wooden handle brush from the supermarket that would normally be used for cleaning vegetables. Like wood, leather has a grain (the direction in which the hide of the animal used to make the leather grew). By looking at your leather, determine which way the grain runs. It is advisable, but not absolutely necessary, to brush the leather with the grain.

After the large particulate material has been removed from your leather, use a product to clean down into its pores. If you want to spend a lot of money, you can always take your leather to the drycleaners. However, there is a much cheaper way to get your leather clean. Many products are available at a wide variety of locations, ranging from Tandy Leather to the local shoe store. These products range in price from a couple of dollars to $25 a bottle. I have found the more reasonably priced products usually work just as well as the expensive ones. Without endorsing a particular product, I will say I prefer to use saddle soap. There are different versions of this product, usually sold in a can like traditional wax shoe polish.

Because of proprietary information, I don't know how the formulae for these products vary, but I have found that they work equally well. Following the directions on the can, use a damp (not wet) sponge or soft cloth to work the soap into a good lather on your leather. (Say *that* three times, fast!) Usually a circular motion will accomplish this, but do not expect the type of foaming that you would see with dish soap. Before the lather has a chance to dry, wipe it off with another clean damp sponge or cloth. Despite some saddle soap manufacturers' directions, never let saddle soap dry on your leather! The result is a dingy finish hard to remove, even with further cleaning. After wiping off the lather, allow the leather to dry slowly as discussed above. When the leather is dry, you can use a soft dry cloth to buff it to a shine. Even if you do not encounter mud or other dirty substances, it is recommended that you clean your leather from time to time thoroughly. (I must point out that saddle soap is not intended to clean suede leather. I will cover the cleaning of suede later in the chapter.)

While regular cleaning is essential for preserving the life of your leather goods, the process of removing dust and dirt also depletes the hide of oils and other conditioners needed to keep the leather soft and to protect it from drying and cracking. Therefore, after each time you clean your leather, you must replenish these emollients. As with cleaning products, there are many apt moisturizers on the market, ranging in price and formulation. Although the formulation may be different, the basic premise is to add moisture to the hide and seal it there to keep it from evaporating and further drying the hide. Find a product that works for you. I prefer to use Lexol Leather Conditioner (this company also produces a cleaner), or even plain Neats Foot Oil. If the product comes in a spray bottle, spray a little at a time and wipe with a clean, soft, cloth until the conditioner is spread lightly and evenly over the leather. If the product does not come in a spray-on formulation, dampen a cloth with it and rub it evenly into the item with a circular motion.

When all surface area has been treated, hang the garment up using a large diameter hanging rod (to avoid creases) and allow the oil to sink into the hide. This will not take much time if the hide is very dry. After a few minutes, return to the garment with another clean, soft cloth and wipe off any excess oil. In the case of leather conditioners, more is not better. Too much conditioner with a lot of oil will clog the pores of your leather. This stops the "breathing" process which allows air in and moisture out. And so a pair of boots, worn often on unusually sweaty feet, may become moldy. Additionally, do not condition your leather unless you have cleaned it first. Conditioning before cleaning will seal in unwanted dirt and grime, causing the leather to age before its time. In addition to conditioning your leather, the oils found in many products also provide natural waterproofing. Of course, never use conditioners not specifically formulated for use on leather items.

In general, suede will become soiled fairly quickly because of its texture. Dark spots caused by grease or other wetting agents will invariably show up first because of the natural attraction dust and dirt have for these substances. Suede requires special treatment, but is fairly simple to take care of as well. After every use, when the item is dry, brush the garment with a stiff brush to remove dust and dirt on the surface. This is essential for preserving a new-looking appearance. If you have a particularly dirty area not produced by a stain, rub it with an artgum eraser. If you get caught in the rain, blot off as much water as you can and then let the garment dry slowly. Then brush as directed above. If the garment has become stained, go to your local leather shop and purchase a cleaner made specifically for suede. Typically, these products are sprayed on, allowed to dry, and the item is then brushed to remove the staining materials loosened by the cleaner. To preserve the nap of the suede, always brush in one direction. Some suede cleaners also come with coloring agents if the offending stain produces discoloration. Before using a suede cleaner, always be sure to test it in an inconspicuous area of the material to make sure that discoloration does not occur.

In addition to suede, there are many specialty leathers on the market today, particularly when it comes to boots. As they are different from cow skin, they often require special treatment. Snake, alligator, lizard, and turtle leather have special membranes that hold the scales together. In order to keep the scales in top condition, leather conditioners must be applied more frequently to leather tanned from hides of these animals. And even though sharkskin is extremely tough and scratch-resistant, it can dry and crack easily. Therefore, it also requires more frequent conditioning.

Always store your leather in a clean, dry place. A damp or warm storage area will invite the growth of unwanted mold and mildew. Unfortunately, many areas of the world have high levels of humidity through most of the year. Some people in these areas, in an attempt to control mildew, store their leather in plastic bags to keep out moisture. This will actually accomplish the opposite affect. Never use tightly sealed storage bags as leather requires freely circulating air. If your household is so humid that you have problems controlling mold and mildew, it may be wise to invest in a dehumidifier. And never store your leather with mothballs or moth-repellent sprays. First of all, I have never heard of a moth that decided to become a carnivore. The chemicals that fight moths may end up discoloring your leather.

As incredible as it may sound, that's all there is to taking great care of your leather. However, to entice you to further reading, the next chapter—remember *Hints From Heloise*—will help you with tricky problems and specialty situations.

HELPFUL LEATHER CARE HINTS

While I was writing this book, it occurred to me that an astute reader might notice an apparent contradiction. On one hand, I have described how leather encounters some harsh conditions and handling; on the other, I have been careful to point out the need for tender loving care. Leather *can* take a lot of abuse. However, as with our own bodies, a lot of TLC must be added between the periods of abuse to ensure long life.

Many people acquire their leather used. While this is a thrifty way to buy what can sometimes be an expensive commodity, it may also result in an item that doesn't fit so well. Also, since leather can last a lifetime with proper care, many owners encounter a middle-age bulge that causes a snug fit. Here are hints to help get your leather to fit better—though don't expect miracles.

Shrinking

If you find your leather item is too large, you may be able to shrink it by the following method. First, be sure to clean and condition the leather as outlined in the previous chapter. Allow the garment to set for a day or so to ensure that the conditioner has had a chance to penetrate deeply. Throw the item into your clothes dryer, set on medium heat, and dry it for about 10 minutes. Take it out and test the level of shrinkage. Repeat this process until the leather fits better. Remember, this will NOT cause a size 44 jacket to turn into a size 38. This will only help with small adjustments. Leather has a tendency to want to retain its shape. Don't be surprised if an item you shrank one time requires further treatment at a later date. After you have finished, don't forget to give the item a final conditioning treatment to help prevent cracking due to the heat treatment.

Many people wear leather chaps when riding horses, or a motorcycle. One of the most common complaints about chaps and leather pants is that they have a tendency to stretch, particularly in the knee. To help these and other trouble areas maintain their shape, break out the iron and ironing board. No, I'm not out of my mind; leather can be ironed. Simply place the leather between two paper bags, or two towels. Set your iron to medium heat and iron away for a couple of minutes, try the garment on for fit, and repeat as necessary. Keep the iron moving to avoid overheating. Don't forget to clean the item before ironing and to condition the leather after treatment to prevent cracking.

Stretching

A somewhat easier process than shrinking is stretching. Many items of leather, from boots to chaps, can be made larger in a relatively short period of time. Like shrinking, you will not be able to obtain a many-fold increase in size, but small adjustments to accommodate normal growth can be obtained.

To stretch your leather, start with a trip to the local leather store for a spray-on product made to stretch leather. As with cleaners and conditioners, there are many brands. It has been my experience that they all work similarly. Following manufacturer's recommendations, spray or rub the chemical into the leather, dosing liberally. The easiest way to ensure that the leather stretches to your size, without overdoing it, is to wear the item for several hours. I must reiterate that if you can't fit into the item to start with, you probably won't get the results you want. Once the item drys out a little, repeat the process if necessary. The leather item may want to shrink over time, but repeated wearing will force it to maintain its increased size. This procedure will work best if the item is not lined with material, but usually these linings will give a little as well.

Linings

Many leather items, especially jackets, shirts and pants, contain some sort of lining so the seams where the leather is joined won't scratch the wearer. Over time, dirt, body oils and sweat stains can cause these linings to become unsightly. If the lining is silk, mix up a dilute solution of Woolite and apply it to the lining with a damp sponge. Remove the detergent by rinsing with a clean, damp sponge. A similar process is used for nylon linings, but use Woolite spray-foam upholstery cleaner. Once the lining has dried, remove the detergent by vacuuming. With today's smaller appliances and attachments, it is not too difficult to reach all areas, especially if the item is turned inside out. Many of today's boot manufacturers use cloth instead of leather for the leg portion of their product. This method may also be used to clean these fabrics as well.

Chrome

Modern leather items also often come with

decorative studs and other metallic adornments. These items are more often than not made of a cheaper metal like nickel, and not chrome, and tend to oxidize with contact to air, and lose their luster. To keep studs looking their best, break out the Windex. Spray lightly and wipe with a paper towel, just as if you were cleaning your windows. Keep in mind that this product does contain alcohol which may release some dye from the leather. To obtain a bright shine to the metal, and to help condition the leather, apply a very light coating of baby oil. Over time the baby oil will also dull, so it is necessary to repeat the process.

Travel

To help avoid creases in your leather garments while traveling, it is best to roll rather than fold them. For example, with a pair of chaps, place the insides of the legs together. Starting from either end, not the long sides, roll the leather loosely until you reach the other end. Simple huh? You may be pleasantly surprised that you can often fit more into one bag this way.

When packing your favorite boots, stuff them with the socks you are going to pack anyway. This not only helps keep the boots from getting crushed, but also gives you extra room to pack.

When including a flogger (many-tailed whip) in your travel plans, wrap the tails around the stiff handle. You can tie them there loosely with a piece of string or a rubber band. This serves two purposes. The tails of the flogger are less likely to become creased or tangled as the bag's contents shift during flight. Longer whips can be coiled around themselves and tied to keep them from becoming tangled as well.

Once at your destination, be sure and unpack as quickly as practical. Hang up all items. Uncoil floggers and allow them to dangle naturally. If you do find that something has become creased during travel, you may iron the spot to help remove the mark. Follow the directions in this chapter.

Disinfection of Whips, Floggers, and other "Toys"

Although this book is meant for the general public, this section is included specifically for those who engage in certain kinds of alternative sexual play, such as SM. Some of these activities can lead to mild or severe skin abrasions which cause leather items to come into contact with body fluids, including blood. In this age of HIV and hepatitis infection, care must be taken to protect those who engage in these activities from inadvertent disease transmission. The following is the generally accepted method for disinfection of non-disposable leather items.

After engaging in any activities that exposes your leather items to body fluids, you must clean and disinfect the items. Even if the skin does not appear to be broken, tiny microabrasions can occur. So, if there's any possibility that your leather came into contact with body fluids, follow these steps.

First, clean the item with soap as outlined in the previous chapter. Because these items come in contact with proteins from the skin, use cold to lukewarm water with the soap. Never use hot water which causes the proteins to coagulate and fix onto the leather item, much in the same way the white of an egg coagulates when cooked. This makes future cleaning very difficult and almost guarantees the item will not be disinfected.

Once the item has dried slowly, treat the leather to kill microorganisms that may be present on the surface, or deep in the pores. Many types of commercial disinfectants could be used for disinfection, including Lysol or household bleach. But the porous nature of leather will cause the chemicals in these to become trapped. If a person's skin is broken the next time leather treated with such disinfectants is used, chemicals could enter the body, with the potential for harmful side-effects, including allergic reactions. So, the best way to disinfect leather is to treat liberally with 70% rubbing (isopropyl) alcohol. Fill a household spray bottle with the alcohol and spray all surfaces. Be generous with the spray to ensure that the alcohol penetrates deep into all crevices. Hang the leather and allow it to dry slowly. The alcohol will evaporate, and so will not affect the next person to come into contact with the leather.

Because leather dyes often have an alcohol base, do not be surprised if some of the leather's color is lost. I will cover re-dyeing below.

You'll find rubbing alcohol in two percentages, 70 and 90. It is important to use 70% for two reasons. First, the small amount of water in the 70% formulation keeps the alcohol from evaporating too quickly. This allows greater contact time between the alcohol and the microorganism (bacteria or viruses), thus allowing for more efficient killing. Secondly, membranes are made of two types of molecules, hydrophobic and hydrophillic. Hydro is the root word meaning water. Phobic means hating. Oils are hydrophobic molecules, thus they do not mix with water. Phyllic is the exact opposite of phobic. The water in the 70% alcohol dissolves the hydrophillic molecules in the membrane, helping the alcohol to work.

In addition to releasing dye from the leather, alcohol will really strip away the conditioners. Once the implement has dried, prevent cracking and splitting by applying a conditioner, as previously outlined. Depending on how much conditioner is lost on a particular application, more than one treatment with Lexol or your favorite brand may be necessary. Be sure to allow the conditioner to penetrate fully into the leather before using on another person. This entire process is not to be rushed. Take your time, to ensure that all surfaces have been cleaned and adequately disinfected.

These same principals should be followed for leather dildoes as well. To the chagrin of every kinky leather store, I'm sure I would like to persuade each of you either to not purchase these items, or to cover them with condoms before every use. Leather dildoes are hard to clean, and inserting dyed leather into anal or vaginal orifices can lead to severe allergic reactions. In addition, the linings of these body parts are very vascular (filled with blood vessels) which allows free diffusion of dyes and chemicals into the blood stream.

Dyeing of Leather

As mentioned above, disinfecting leather can lead to the release of dye. Most quality leathers are heavily impregnated with excess dye and a few treatments with alcohol will not be enough to significantly discolor them. Lower quality leather and those of lighter weight will naturally lose their coloration more quickly. And many people often wish to change the color of their leather, most commonly from natural (brown) to black.

Leather dyeing means another trip to your local shoe repair shop or leather store, where small bottles of leather dye can be purchased. Again, follow the manufacturers' directions while keeping the following in mind. You may want to invest in a pair of rubber gloves to avoid dyeing your hands. Always practice dyeing on scrap leather, so you will become familiar with the dye and its application without ruining your good leathers. To avoid streaking and to ensure evenness in dye uptake, clean and dry your leather thoroughly before adding pigment. Place the leather on a clean, absorbent material. Newspapers or cardboard are excellent. When applying the dye, move the applicator back and forth from one end of the piece of leather to the other, or move it in a circular motion, overlapping previous strokes as you progress from one end to the other. To avoid streaking, and to create even tone, overlap your strokes on each pass. I find the circular motion works best. Do not be surprised if one area of the leather takes more dye than others. This is natural, depending on the grain. After you have completely dyed the leather, allow it to dry for a few minutes. Then go back and repeat the process. Several applications will be needed to penetrate the leather deeply, and this will also help maintain an even dye appearance. Don't try to apply one heavy coat, as you will just be disappointed in the end result. When dyeing from a light color to a dark color, use intermediate colors. For example, when dyeing from brown to black, start off by giving the leather a couple of coats of blue dye. After this is applied, move onto the black. This method will also help to promote evenness of color. These processes take time, so for best results don't rush.

Once the dye has set into the leather, seal it there with a process called *finishing*. Dyes will also have a tendency to dry leather, so in addition to helping the leather hold the dye, this process also conditions it as well. Many commercial finishing products are available, but I have had good luck using my normal conditioner, Lexol. If you happen to get dye on metal adornments of the leather, use a Q-tip and a little alcohol to remove it.

A SHORT HISTORY OF RUBBER

There are many different rubbers each with its own chemical formula and properties. In this chapter, I am discussing latex rubber, both natural and man-made. And science buffs might want to know that latex rubber, *cis*-1,4-polyisoprene, has the chemical formula $(C_5H_8)n$.

Though latex is produced naturally by nearly 2,000 species of trees, shrubs and vines in temperate and tropical regions, the only significant commercial sources are plantations of the tree *Hevea brasiliensis*. Although cultivated around the world, this tree is indigenous to the Amazon valley.

Inhabitants of South America have known of rubber for centuries, but Christopher Columbus was probably the first European to handle it. During his second voyage (1493-1496), Columbus noted that natives played a game with elastic balls made of a substance obtained from trees they called cau-uhu. In approximately 1615, useful applications of the substance were described by Juan de Torquemada. He gave an accounting of the waterproofing of clothing by natives of Mexico, with a substance they called ulei, extracted from the ule tree.

The word "rubber" was coined by John Priestly in 1770, when he discovered that this material could erase pencil marks. European interest in rubber was not piqued until two French scientists, La Condamine and Fresneau, made further observations. During a scientific trip to the equator, La Condamine sent samples to the Academy of Sciences. This dark, resin-like substance was extracted from the heve tree by cutting into the bark. At first, a white milky liquid, like sap, flowed from the tree. However, upon exposure to air, the substance solidified and turned dark. Fresneau met La Condamine in 1743 and it was he who first described the rubber tree in detail, including how it was grown and how to obtain rubber from it.

It was not long before it was discovered that other plants were capable of producing the same material. By the end of the 18th century, Europe and America were using only a few tons of rubber a year.

This low usage could be attributed to the difficulty experienced when working with the solid material. Items made from the material became stiff in cold temperatures and very sticky when exposed to heat.

It wasn't until the 19th century that technology had advanced enough to solve these problems, allowing the rubber industry to become a multibillion dollar operation. Thomas Hancock observed that freshly cut pieces of rubber, when put in contact with one another, would stick together. He came up with the idea of chopping these pieces finely then reforming them into any desired shape or size. He produced a machine called the masticator that ground, softened, mixed and shaped solid rubber. Instead of producing a powder as expected, this machine converted the hard, elastic rubber into a pasty, plastic mass that could be molded, and he also found the mess took up dry chemicals in great quantity.

Rubber was still limited in use due to the economic losses encountered by all companies who endeavored to use it. Rubber articles in perfect condition when they left factories would rapidly deteriorate and become sticky when exposed to light and heat. They also still became hard and brittle when exposed to cold. Indeed, mastication actually contributed to the decline in the rubber industry.

The full impact in the importance of mastication was not discovered until the work of one man, Charles Goodyear. In 1831, he started experiments to improve upon the properties of rubber, including a "drier" which would prevent the stickiness when exposed to heat. In 1839, he came up with the process of vulcanization. He found that if crude rubber was mixed with sulphur above the melting point of the latter, it would more easily withstand changes in temperature. Since that time, the manufacturing processes of modern rubber have included ingredients to confer rubber with many different properties. These ingredients and processes include acceleration of vulcanization, the use of antioxidants, and reinforcing fillers.

After Goodyear's breakthrough, the demand for rubber products grew rapidly. Exports of raw rubber from Brazil multiplied almost 100-fold from 1846 to 1880. Until this explosion in demand, all raw rubber was supplied to the industry from naturally occurring plants. Soon however, demand far exceeded supply. The British were the first to consider the cultivation of rubber in Asia. In 1876, Henry Wickham collected seeds from Brazil for cultivation. From the seeds that germinated, some plants went to Sri Lanka and others to Singapore and Malaysia. Later, other plants were sent to Indonesia (note modern names used). By 1880, the *Hevea* seedlings were widely distributed in Asia.

Also helping meet demand was the work of Henry Ridley, who while in Singapore in the 1890's devised a more effective and economical method for extracting raw latex. His method, called *tapping*, caused less damage to the tree and yielded greater quantities.

The use of acid to coagulate, concentrate and produce sheets of latex, which were then dried in smoke, was discovered by John Perkins in 1899. Before that time in 1888, John Dunlop increased demand for this product by his invention of the pneumatic tire (a tube filled with air).

The production of plantation rubber in Asia grew rapidly. By 1913 most rubber was produced in this fashion. To this day, Southeast Asia is the predominant region for rubber cultivation.

Although scientists tried to produce a synthetic substitute for natural latex, most chemical reactions produced a product with altered chemistry, and therefore altered characteristics. It was only during World War I that Germany, cut off from every country exporting natural rubber, was able to synthesize methyl rubber, with the same basic properties as nature's own rubber. After the war, production was abandoned because of high cost, but small-scale research continued. Demand for synthetic rubbers also rose during World War II, when many types of synthetic rubbers, still in use today, were discovered. However, they often are used for very specific purposes, from specialty tires to machine gaskets and protective clothing with resistance to hazardous chemicals. It wasn't until 1955 that American researchers were able to produce polyisoprene (latex) rubber. Since that time, companies in other countries have begun the production of this substance. However, it is still more economically feasible to acquire latex rubber from natural sources.

THE PROCESSING OF RAW LATEX RUBBER

This chapter offers an overview of the processing of latex. The steps are involved and complex, often including many chemical additives. There is no way all of the information could be included in this book.

Previously mentioned was the fact that latex is produced from plantations of the *Hevea* tree. The latex is contained in a network of capillary tubes, which exist in all parts of the tree. These vessels form a continuous network much like the blood vessels of mammals. These vessels form vertical bundles arranged in a fairly regular pattern around the trunk of the tree. Latex is obtained from latex vessels in the tree by *tapping*, a process similar to that used to obtain sap for the production of maple syrup. Tapping occurs before sunrise, when the greatest pressure exists in the latex vessels. Three to four hours after tapping, the raw latex is collected and treated to prevent premature coagulation. The material is sent to a processing center where ammonia, sodium sulfite or formaldehyde is added as a stabilizer.

At the factory, huge vats of latex are diluted to bring the rubber content to about 20 percent. Note that raw rubber also contains other substances including proteins, lipids (fat), carbohydrates and inorganic (not containing carbon) molecules. The latex is put into large vats with aluminum partitions. Acetic or formic acid is added to the latex to induce coagulation. Coagulation occurs around the partitions to form sheets. These gelatinous slabs are compressed through wringers to remove water and produce sheets of uniform thickness. From this point on, any number of processes may occur. The rubber sheets can be dried for 4-7 days in smoke houses, keeping the sheets at about 60 degrees Celsius (140 degrees Fahrenheit) by burning wood. Alternately, the sheets may be dried by a current of hot air, without the use of smoke. The dried sheets are packed into bales coated with talc to prevent adhesion from bale to bale. Many other processes occur including vulcanization, addition of fillers, and compounding agents which change the physical properties of the latex, depending on its final use from tires to clothing. Processes may also occur to remove the non-latex portions of the raw rubber. Which processes occur depend on the final destination and intended use of the latex, and are too numerous to discuss adequately here.

THE CARE OF LATEX GARMENTS

Latex is one of the most interesting "fabrics" produced today. In addition to its visual appeal, latex often provides the wearer with many new inputs for the senses. Unlike other fabrics, latex garments are typically worn tight, and so do not rub against the body like most clothing. This leads to a somewhat diminished sense of touch. Latex garments cause the body to heat surprisingly quickly in warm weather, and allow the wearer to lose body heat in colder climates. Latex also has a particular odor. All of these factors, and more, lead to a (if you will pardon the cliche) feast for the senses—not only for the wearer, but also for passersby.

Before you rush out to your latex-wear, there are some health concerns to garments made of latex. Why? Because natural rubber latex is a plant material and as such may induce allergic reactions in certain individuals. Even if a person is not allergic to the natural properties of latex, allergies can develop to the additives used during processing. In the age of AIDS, where condoms and rubber gloves are being used more frequently, the incidence of allergic reactions is increasing. Allergic reactions may be as mild as sneezing and watering eyes, or they may actually induce anaphylactic shock, characterized by shortness of breath, swollen lips and heart palpitations, and death if not treated immediately. People allergic to bee stings will know what I mean.

One must be aware that we are not necessarily born with allergies. They can develop over a period of months. I know of no way, short of actual use, to determine if a person is allergic to latex. However, if you have been using condoms or latex gloves for a long time without symptoms, it should be okay for you to don latex garments. If statistics are your bag: according to an Associated Press article, seven percent of surgeons and five percent of operating room nurses had become allergic to the latex in their surgical gloves. If you develop an allergy, see your doctor, or in the case of anaphylactic shock, call 911.

Once you have determined that you will not be subjected to any unwanted discomfort due to wearing latex garments, you are now set to spend your hard-earned dollars. Be aware that latex, like leather, can be expensive and of differing quality. If you see two similar items at two different shops, with greatly varying prices, check to make sure they are actually the same. Many latex items are constructed from sheets of latex, cut in a pattern, and glued together. While they may appear to be identical, upon closer examination you may find that they were fabricated from latex sheets of different thicknesses. You will most often find that thicker sheets are more resistant to tears. Other garments may be manufactured by a molding process, and often these items come from only one source. Also, be aware that many shops catering to the latex enthusiast will not allow you to try on clothing before purchase. Often, one must adjust sizes to account for stretching, tightness and personal preferences. If at all possible, hook up with a friend who may have a similar item. Try it on and compare for fit. Obviously, a large man will not fit into a small latex shirt, so try and pick a friend who is close to your size.

The first rule to taking care of your latex is to avoid sharp objects. A major contributor to early puncture wounds to latex items is the dreaded finger, in particular the finger's nail. Be sure to trim them before putting on your latex. Also be sure to remove all jewelry that may be raised. Most jewelry used for body piercing will be okay to use with latex garments, but take care nonetheless.

Unless lubricated in some fashion, latex garments naturally possess a high degree of friction. In an analogous fashion to rubber car tires stopping on pavement, latex garments can tear on flat surfaces. You rub against a wall and keep walking, but the rubber stops. Without enough give, or loosened contact, the rubber will tear.

If you do happen to tear your garment, don't despair—it can probably be repaired. Many producers of latex garments offer a repair service. Call them in advance to determine if this is the case. If tears or punctures are minor, you may be able to make your own repairs. This is where scraps of latex come in handy. Often, scraps can be purchased, but you should save any articles of latex-wear damaged beyond repair. Go to your local sporting goods dealer and buy an inner-tube repair kit. Cut a patch from the scrap latex to fit over the hole or tear. Turn the damaged item inside out. Using the "roughing tool" usually supplied in the tire repair kit, rough up the edges around the hole. Also rough up the edges of the patch. Apply glue liberally, but not so much that excess oozes from around the patch. Allow the glue to set for a few minutes, then cement the seal with some pressure. I put the item between two sheets of plastic wrap to avoid getting glue everywhere, and then use a large book on a flat surface to provide steady pressure until the glue has completely set. Excess glue can often be removed by using a pencil eraser, being careful not to re-tear the garment. This usually doesn't work well for unusually large holes, but it does work fine for those minor emergencies.

When putting on your latex garment, be sure to give all internal surfaces a good dusting with powder. Many people use baby powder, but I prefer to use plain talc since it is unscented. I have also been known to use Gold Bond Medicated Powder. This works great, especially if one is prone to jock itch. The medicine in the powder alleviates itching associated with sweating around the groin. Of course, this does not work if one uses lubricant inside the garment for that slippery feeling. Be aware that this particular powder has oils which may damage latex in the long run. I will discuss oils and lubricants more in a following section.

Latex has a normally dull appearance, but many people prefer to shine it. Any number of products are useful for this purpose, but the polishing agent must be not only water soluble, but also water based. Because latex and oils are both hydrocarbons (complex molecules of hydrogen and carbon) any oil-based compound used on latex will cause it to disintegrate. Black Beauty (a product made specifically for latex clothing), Turtle Wax Clearguard, and food safe KingCo Silicone Spray all work well. Before using any new product, be sure to test it on a small scrap of latex. Before applying the polishing agent, use a damp cloth to wipe off any talcum powder on the outside surface. When wiping either to clear talcum or to apply a polishing agent, be sure to use a cloth that is free from lint, or you may appear speckled under the black light found in many establishments. Again, be sure that only water-based lubricants are used to give that slippery feel inside the latex, if you are so inclined while wearing it. And never insert any latex that has been polished with the above products into any body orifice, including the vagina and anus.

Taking off latex can be an adventure in itself. It is best to ease the garment off, especially if very tight, by rolling or turning the garment inside-out while removing it. Be careful not to grab with your nails. Be especially careful when removing latex items like t-shirts over your head, especially if it is tight to begin with. Latex has the ability to form an air-tight seal that rivals Tupperware. Many people recommend that removing latex in a warm (not hot) shower is easier. Be careful when doing this as the latex can still form a seal and you could drown if the garment fills with running water. This sounds drastic, but when one comes home alone after a long night at a favorite watering hole...

After every use, clean your latex thoroughly. You may think that it isn't dirty, but body oils, or the likes of Crisco, can doom your latex. To clean, fill a sink or bathtub with warm water. Squirt in some mild liquid dish soap. Use a clean cloth to gently wash all surfaces. I prefer to use Ivory Brand dish soap. It is closest to pure soap and among the mildest. Most other brands of dish soaps (especially Dawn) and laundry detergents contain harsh grease-cutting agents which ensure your favorite fry pan comes clean, but which will also eat into your latex. Remember that oil and latex are chemically similar. One friend of mine used Dawn on one occasion and found his latex was sticky the next day. Also, never use abrasive cleaners on your latex. Once you have cleaned all surfaces of the garment, be sure to rinse it well and hang it to dry. Often you will find creases or internal surfaces to be wet after initial drying. Turn the item to the other side out and complete drying. Once the item is completely dry, dust it with talcum powder and store it.

Storage of latex usually takes two forms—hanging them in a cool, dry closet or rolling (not folding them) and storing them in large plastic bags in a drawer. Always keep your latex away from excess light and heat. Many people hang their leather and latex in the same closet or wear them together. Be careful when doing so. The emollients used to condition leather can eat through latex. I learned this lesson the hard way. I had a latex shirt hanging in my leather closet. I usually kept them separated, but one day I didn't pay attention when hanging the shirt. A few days later, when I planned to wear the shirt, I found that a small hole had sprouted. What had happened? My latex shirt had brushed against leather. After cursing at myself for my carelessness, I stashed the shirt back in the closet, planning to use the undamaged portions for future repairs needs. Oops—more carelessness. When I went back into the closet after about two months, all I found was a heap of black ooze on the floor. The leather-dressing residue on the leather clothing had acted as a catalyst to destroy the latex. The lesson to be learned is to take care of your latex promptly if oil-based substances come into contact with it. So—be careful when mixing leather and latex garments.

Other things to keep in mind are that the ultraviolet light (UV) found in sunlight will cause your latex to appear streaked and will ultimately lead to its demise. Never dry your latex by artificial means. You could end up with a sticky mess like I found at the bottom of my closet. There is one exception to this drying rule. Many people who store their latex in drawers will find that creases can develop. To eliminate these, simply hang the item up and allow the creases to be "ironed" out by the weight of the garment. If a crease is especially bad, the following method can be used if *extreme* care is taken. Hang the item on a clothes hanger. Using an electric hair dryer (blow dryer) on a low setting, carefully and quickly move the dryer so that heat is evenly applied to the crease. Be careful not to leave the dryer in one place too long or you will end up burning a hole!

If you remember that latex requires more caution and care than leather, you will find it to be fantastically fun, and an eye catching garment.

CONCLUSION

As stated previously, this book is to be used as a general primer for leather and latex care. Many fine products too numerous to mention are available to clean and condition your leather. With a little trial, and hopefully no error, you will find the one you like best. The best way to take care of your leather, whether it is old and worn or brand new, is to keep it clean and conditioned. Store in a cool, dry place. Leather is meant to last a lifetime and even under adverse conditions it will last longer than other fabrics.

Latex is much more delicate and requires closer attention than leather. Always dust your latex with talcum powder—to wear and to store. Clean your latex with mild soap (no grease-cutters) after every use. Only use water-based lubricants with your latex. Avoid exposure to sunlight, sharp objects, and excessive heat.

I hope you have found this book to be helpful. In addition to being helpful, I also hope you will find leather and latex care to be a fairly simple task. Best of luck with these two "wonder garments."

ABOUT THE AUTHOR

Kelly J. Thibault was born and raised in a small town in Montana to parents of "good peasant stock." Some of his earliest and fondest memories are of times spent at his father's shoe repair shop. He left home to attend college and now holds his M.S. in biological sciences with an emphasis in molecular genetics, useful for his current career in the biotechnology industry.

Mr. Thibault is well known in the leather and SM communities. He held the title of Mr. Orange Coast Drummer '91, was the author of Leather Rap, a newspaper column covering leather community news and events, was founder of the leather/SM educational group Orange Coast Leather Assembly, and was also the founder of SandMen, a leather/SM educational and social organization. He has also lectured and presented workshops on a variety of leather/SM-related topics at universities, conferences, community events and organization meetings.

Carried Away

An s/M Romance

In david stein's first novel, steamy Leathersex is only the beginning when a cocky, jaded bottom and a once-burned Master come together for some no-strings bondage and S/M. Once the scene is over, a deeper hunger unexpectedly awakens, and they begin playing for much higher stakes.

$19.95

Ties That Bind

The SM/Leather/Fetish Erotic Style
Issues, Commentaries and Advice

The early writings of well-known psychotherapist and respected member of the leather community Guy Baldwin have been compiled to create this SM classic. Second edition. **$16.95**

SlaveCraft

Roadmaps for Erotic Servitude Principles, Skills and Tools

Guy Baldwin, author of *Ties That Bind*, joins forces with a grateful slave to produce this gripping and personal account on the subject of consensual slavery. **$15.95**

The Master's Manual

A Handbook of Erotic Dominance

In this book, author Jack Rinella examines various aspects of erotic dominance, including S/M, safety, sex, erotic power, techniques and more. The author speaks in a clear, frank, and nonjudgmental way to anyone with an interest in the erotic Dominant/submissive dynamic. **$15.95**

The Compleat Slave

Creating and Living and Erotic Dominant/submissive Lifestyle

In this highly anticipated follow up to The Master's Manual, author Jack Rinella continues his in-depth exploration of Dominant/submissive relationships. **$15.95**

Learning the Ropes

A Basic Guide to Fun S/M Lovemaking

This book, by S/M expert Race Bannon, guides the reader through the basics of safe and fun S/M. Negative myths are dispelled and replaced with the truth about the kind of S/M erotic play that so many adults enjoy. **$12.95**

My Private Life

Real Experiences of a Dominant Woman

Within these pages, the author, Mistress Nan, allows the reader a brief glimpse into the true private life of an erotically dominant woman. Each scene is vividly detailed and reads like the finest erotica, but knowing that these scenes really occurred as written adds to the sexual excitement they elicit. Second Edition. **$16.95**

Consensual Sadomasochism

How to Talk About It and How to Do It Safely

Authors William A. Henkin, Ph. D. and Sybil Holiday, CCHT combine their extensive professional credentials with deep personal experience in this unique examination of erotic consensual sadomasochism. Second edition. **$17.95**

Chainmale: 3SM

A Unique View of Leather Culture

Author Don Bastian brings his experiences to print with this fast paced account of one man's experience with his own sexuality and eventual involvement in a loving and successful three-way kink relationship. **$13.95**

Leathersex

A Guide for the Curious Outsider and the Serious Player

Written by renowned S/M author Joseph Bean, this book gives guidance to one popular style of erotic play which the author calls 'leathersex'- sexuality that may include S/M, bondage, role playing, sensual physical stimulation and fetish, to name just a few. Second edition. **$16.95**

Leathersex Q&A

Questions About Leathersex and the Leather Lifestyle Answered

In this interesting and informative book, author Joseph Bean answers a wide variety of questions about leathersex sexuality. Each response is written with the sensitivity and insight only someone with a vast amount of experience in this style of sexuality could provide. **$16.95**

Beneath The Skins

The New Spirit and Politics of the Kink Community

This book by Ivo Dominguez, Jr. examines the many issues facing the modern leather/SM/fetish community. This special community is coming of age, and this book helps to pave the way for all who are a part of it. **$12.95**

Between The Cracks

The Daedalus Anthology of Kinky Verse

Editor Gavin Dillard has collected the most exotic of the erotic of the poetic pantheon, from the fetishes of Edna St. Vincent Millay to the howling of Ginsberg, lest any further clues be lost *between the cracks*. **$18.95**

The Leather Contest Guide

A Handbook for Promoters, Contestants, Judges and Titleholders

International Mr. Leather and Mr. National Leather Association contest winner Guy Baldwin is the author of this truly complete guide to the leather contest. Second Edition. **$14.95**

Ordering Information

Phone
323.666.2121

Email
info@DaedalusPublishing.com

Mail
Daedalus Publishing Company, 2140 Hyperion Ave, Los Angeles, CA 90027

Payment

All major credit cards are accepted. Via *email or regular mail*, indicate type of card, card number, expiration date, name of cardholder as shown on card, and billing address of the cardholder. Also include the mailing address where you wish your order to be sent. Orders via regular mail may include payment by money order or check, but may be held until the check clears. Make checks or money orders payable to "Daedalus Publishing Company." *Do not send cash*.

Tax and shipping

California residents, add 8.25% sales tax to the total price of the books you are ordering. *All* orders should include a $4.25 shipping charge for the first book, plus $1.00 for each additional book added to the total of the order.

Over 21 Statement
Since many of our publications deal with sexuality issues, please include a signed statement that you are at least 21 years of age with any order. Also include such a statement with any email order.